BLOOD TYPE AB-POSITIVE DIET BOOK

"Delicious Recipes and a Complete Guide for your Blood Type for Maximum Wellness"

Dayna G. Murphy

Copyright © 2024 by Dayna G. Murphy
All rights reserved.

Disclaimer: The information provided in this book is for educational purposes only and is not intended as a substitute for professional medical advice, diagnosis, or treatment.

GAIN ACCESS TO OTHER BOOKS BY ME

TABLE OF CONTENTS

INTRODUCTION

"Growing up with my blood type, I always felt a unique connection to the foods that resonated with my body. I struggled with digestive issues until I discovered the power of aligning my diet with my blood type. This cookbook is not just a collection of recipes; it's a journey of self-discovery and a celebration of the incredible impact that food can have on our well-being."

Understanding Blood Type Diets:

Concept of Blood Type Diets:

Blood type diets are based on the idea that individuals with different blood types (A, B, AB, O) should follow specific dietary patterns that align with their genetic makeup. The concept was popularized by a scientist, who proposed that blood types influence how our bodies react to certain foods, impacting overall health and well-being.

Why Blood Type Diets Matter:

The theory suggests that by eating foods compatible with one's blood type, individuals can optimize digestion, enhance energy levels, and reduce the risk of various health issues. The diet is tailored to the unique characteristics associated with each blood type, including genetic predispositions and vulnerabilities.

Benefits of Eating According to Blood Type AB Positive:

1. Improved Digestion:

- The diet emphasizes foods that are easily digestible for Blood Type AB Positive individuals, potentially reducing digestive issues.

2. Enhanced Energy Levels:

- By consuming foods that complement the body's metabolic processes, individuals may experience increased energy and vitality.

3. Weight Management:

- The diet aims to address factors influencing weight gain specific to blood type AB Positive, potentially aiding in weight management.

4. Immune System Support:

- Certain foods are believed to strengthen the immune system, offering protection against illnesses and promoting overall health.

5. Optimal Nutrient Absorption:

- The diet focuses on foods that align with the nutritional needs of Blood Type AB Positive individuals, facilitating better nutrient absorption.

CHAPTER 1: UNDERSTANDING BLOOD TYPE AB POSITIVE DIETS

Brief Overview of Blood Types and Their Characteristics:

1. Blood Type A:

- **Characteristics:** Considered to be more cooperative, sensitive, and adaptable.
- **Diet:** Thrives on a vegetarian-based diet with limited animal protein.

2. Blood Type B:

- **Characteristics:** Seen as independent, creative, and adaptable.
- **Diet:** Benefits from a varied diet including meat, dairy, and vegetables.

3. Blood Type AB:

- **Characteristics:** A mix of A and B traits, often described as rational, calm, and sociable.
- **Diet:** A balanced diet that incorporates elements of both A and B diets.

4. Blood Type O:

- **Characteristics:** Typically described as outgoing, ambitious, and self-confident.

- **Diet:** Flourishes on a high-protein diet, often including meat and seafood.

Specifics of Blood Type AB Positive: Traits, Tendencies, and Health Considerations:

1. Traits:

- **Adaptability:** Blood Type AB Positive individuals are often adaptable, able to navigate various social situations with ease.

- **Rationality:** Known for their rational and analytical thinking.

- **Sociability:** Generally considered sociable and capable of maintaining diverse social connections.

2. Tendencies:

- **Balanced Perspective:** May have a balanced perspective, combining creativity with a logical approach.

- **Open-mindedness:** Tends to be open-minded and willing to explore new ideas.

- **Empathy:** Often empathetic, understanding the feelings and perspectives of others.

3. Health Considerations:

- **Potential for Stress Sensitivity:** Blood Type AB Positive individuals might have a tendency to be more sensitive to stress, impacting overall well-being.

- **Immune System Challenges:** Some individuals may face challenges related to the immune system, emphasizing the importance of a diet that supports immune health.

- **Balanced Exercise:** Engaging in a mix of exercises, including both calming activities (like yoga) and more dynamic exercises, may be beneficial.

Understanding the unique traits, tendencies, and health considerations of Blood Type AB Positive is essential for tailoring a diet that aligns with their specific needs. While the blood type diet is a concept that lacks robust scientific backing, it provides a framework for individuals to explore dietary choices that may enhance their overall health and well-being. Always consult with a healthcare professional before making significant changes to your diet.

CHAPTER 2: GROCERY SHOPPING GUIDE

Foods Beneficial for Blood Type AB Positive Individuals:

1. Proteins:

- **Fish:** Salmon, mackerel, trout.
- **Dairy:** Yogurt, kefir, goat cheese.
- **Eggs:** Rich in protein and versatile.

2. Grains:

- **Rice:** Brown rice, basmati rice.
- **Oats:** Whole oats, oat bran.

3. Fruits:

- **Berries:** Blueberries, cherries, blackberries.
- **Plums:** Provide antioxidants and fiber.

4. Vegetables:

- **Leafy Greens:** Spinach, kale, collard greens.
- **Cruciferous Vegetables:** Broccoli, cauliflower, Brussels sprouts.

5. Legumes:

- **Lentils:** High in protein and fiber.

- **Garbanzo Beans (Chickpeas):** Versatile and nutritious.

6. Nuts and Seeds:

- **Almonds:** Rich in healthy fats and protein.
- **Flaxseeds:** Good source of omega-3 fatty acids.

7. Oils:

- **Olive Oil:** Extra virgin olive oil for cooking and dressings.
- **Flaxseed Oil:** High in omega-3 fatty acids.

8. Beverages:

- **Green Tea:** Contains antioxidants and offers various health benefits.
- **Water:** Hydration is essential for overall health.

9. Spices and Herbs:

- **Turmeric:** Known for its anti-inflammatory properties.
- **Ginger:** Adds flavor and has potential health benefits.

10. Sweeteners:

- **Agave Nectar:** A natural sweetener with a lower glycemic index.

Tips for Selecting Fresh and Organic Ingredients:

1. Choose Local and Seasonal:

- Opt for produce that is in-season and sourced locally for freshness and flavor.

2. Go Organic When Possible:

- Select organic fruits and vegetables to minimize exposure to pesticides and chemicals.

3. Check Labels:

- Read labels carefully, especially for packaged items, and choose products with minimal additives and preservatives.

4. Farmers' Markets and Co-ops:

- Explore farmers' markets and co-ops for a variety of fresh, locally sourced ingredients.

5. Inspect Freshness:

- Examine fruits and vegetables for firmness, vibrant colors, and lack of blemishes or wilting.

6. Consider Sustainable Options:

- Choose seafood that is sustainably sourced to support environmental conservation efforts.

7. Opt for Whole Foods:

- Prioritize whole, unprocessed foods to maximize nutritional content and minimize artificial additives.

8. Use Fresh Herbs:

- Include fresh herbs for flavor and additional nutrients instead of relying solely on salt and processed seasonings.

9. Bulk Buying for Staples:

- Purchase pantry staples like grains, legumes, and nuts in bulk to reduce packaging waste and ensure a constant supply.

10. Mindful Cooking Practices:

- Employ cooking methods that preserve the nutritional content of ingredients, such as steaming or roasting.

By incorporating these foods and tips into the diet, Blood Type AB Positive individuals can create a balanced and nourishing eating plan that aligns with the principles of the blood type diet while focusing on fresh, organic, and whole food choices.

CHAPTER 3: BLOOD TYPE AB+ RECOMMENDED FOODS

BEANS AND LEGUMES

Bean/Legume	Portion Size	Frequency per Week
Lentils	1/2 cup cooked	2-3 times
Garbanzo Beans	1/2 cup cooked	2-3 times
Black Beans	1/2 cup cooked	1-2 times
Navy Beans	1/2 cup cooked	1-2 times
Adzuki Beans	1/2 cup cooked	1-2 times
Pinto Beans	1/2 cup cooked	1-2 times
Cannellini Beans	1/2 cup cooked	1-2 times
Mung Beans	1/2 cup cooked	2-3 times

Notes:

- Portion sizes are based on cooked beans.
- The suggested frequency per week is a general guideline and can be adjusted based on individual preferences and dietary needs.
- It's essential to soak and cook beans properly to enhance digestibility blnd nutrient absorption.

MEAT AND POULTRY

Meat/Poultry	Portion Size	Frequency per Week
Lamb	3-4 ounces cooked	1-2 times
Turkey	3-4 ounces cooked	2-3 times
Rabbit	3-4 ounces cooked	1-2 times
Venison	3-4 ounces cooked	1-2 times
Turkey Bacon	Limited quantities	1-2 times

Notes:

- Portion sizes are based on cooked meat/poultry.
- The suggested frequency per week is a general guideline and can be adjusted based on individual preferences and dietary needs.
- It's advisable to choose lean cuts of meat and poultry and practice healthy cooking methods, such as grilling, baking, or broiling.
- Incorporating a variety of protein sources, including plant-based options, can contribute to a well-balanced diet.

DAIRY AND EGGS

Dairy and Eggs	Portion Size	Frequency per Week
Goat Cheese	1 ounce	2-3 times
Mozzarella Cheese	1 ounce	2-3 times
Feta Cheese	1 ounce	2-3 times
Ricotta Cheese	1/4 cup	1-2 times
Eggs (Organic)	2 eggs	3-4 times
Yogurt (Goat Milk)	1 cup	3-4 times
Kefir (Goat Milk)	1 cup	3-4 times

Notes:

- Portion sizes are based on typical serving sizes for dairy and eggs.

- The suggested frequency per week is a general guideline and can be adjusted based on individual preferences and dietary needs.

- Choose organic and high-quality dairy products, especially if available.

SEAFOODS

Seafood	Portion Size	Frequency per Week
Salmon	3-4 ounces cooked	2-3 times
Mackerel	3-4 ounces cooked	1-2 times
Trout	3-4 ounces cooked	1-2 times
Sardines	3-4 ounces cooked	1-2 times
Halibut	3-4 ounces cooked	1-2 times
Red Snapper	3-4 ounces cooked	1-2 times
Cod	3-4 ounces cooked	1-2 times

Notes:

- Portion sizes are based on cooked seafood.

- The suggested frequency per week is a general guideline and can be adjusted based on individual preferences and dietary needs.

- Choose wild-caught and sustainably sourced seafood whenever possible.

NUTS AND SEEDS

Nuts and Seeds	Portion Size	Frequency per Week
Almonds	1/4 cup	3-4 times
Walnuts	1/4 cup	2-3 times
Flaxseeds	1 tablespoon	3-4 times
Chia Seeds	1 tablespoon	3-4 times
Sunflower Seeds	1/4 cup	2-3 times
Pumpkin Seeds	1/4 cup	2-3 times
Cashews	1/4 cup	1-2 times

Notes:

- Portion sizes are based on typical serving sizes for nuts and seeds.

- The suggested frequency per week is a general guideline and can be adjusted based on individual preferences and dietary needs.

- Choose raw and unsalted nuts and seeds for optimal health benefits.

GRAINS AND CEREALS

Grains and Cereals	Portion Size	Frequency per Week
Rice (Brown/Basmati)	1/2 cup cooked	3-4 times
Oats (Whole Oats)	1/2 cup cooked	3-4 times
Spelt	1/2 cup cooked	2-3 times
Millet	1/2 cup cooked	2-3 times
Quinoa	1/2 cup cooked	2-3 times
Buckwheat	1/2 cup cooked	2-3 times
Amaranth	1/2 cup cooked	2-3 times

Notes:

- Portion sizes are based on typical serving sizes for grains and cereals.
- The suggested frequency per week is a general guideline and can be adjusted based on individual preferences and dietary needs.
- Choose whole grains for higher fiber content and nutritional value.

BEVERAGES

Beverages	Portion Size	Frequency per Week
Green Tea	1-2 cups	Daily
Peppermint Tea	1-2 cups	3-4 times
Ginger Tea	1-2 cups	3-4 times
Hibiscus Tea	1-2 cups	2-3 times
Rooibos Tea	1-2 cups	2-3 times
Water	8-10 cups (8 oz.)	Daily
Herbal Infusions (e.g., Chamomile)	1-2 cups	2-3 times
Coffee (if desired)	1-2 cups	2-3 times

Notes:

- Portion sizes are based on typical serving sizes for beverages.
- The suggested frequency per week is a general guideline and can be adjusted based on individual preferences and tolerance.

FRUITS

Fruits	Portion Size	Frequency per Week
Berries (Blueberries, Strawberries)	1/2 to 1 cup	3-4 times
Plums	1 medium	2-3 times
Cherries	1/2 to 1 cup	2-3 times
Pineapple	1/2 to 1 cup	1-2 times
Grapefruit	1 medium	2-3 times
Kiwi	1-2 medium	2-3 times
Papaya	1/2 to 1 cup	2-3 times

Notes:

- Portion sizes are based on typical serving sizes for fruits.

- The suggested frequency per week is a general guideline and can be adjusted based on individual preferences and dietary needs.

- Including a variety of fruits in different colors can provide a broad spectrum of nutrients.

HERBS AND SPICES

Herbs and Spices	Portion Size	Frequency per Week
Turmeric	1/4 to 1/2 teaspoon	2-3 times
Ginger	1/4 to 1/2 teaspoon	2-3 times
Cilantro	1 tablespoon	3-4 times
Rosemary	1/2 to 1 teaspoon	2-3 times
Thyme	1/2 to 1 teaspoon	2-3 times
Basil	1/4 to 1/2 teaspoon	3-4 times
Dill	1/4 to 1/2 teaspoon	3-4 times
Mint	1 tablespoon	2-3 times

Notes:

- Portion sizes are based on typical usage in cooking.
- The suggested frequency per week is a general guideline and can be adjusted based on individual preferences and dietary needs.
- Experimenting with a variety of herbs and spices can enhance the flavor of meals without relying on excessive salt or unhealthy seasonings.

VEGETABLES

Vegetables	Portion Size	Frequency per Week
Spinach	1 cup raw or 1/2 cup cooked	3-4 times
Kale	1 cup raw or 1/2 cup cooked	2-3 times
Collard Greens	1 cup raw or 1/2 cup cooked	2-3 times
Broccoli	1 cup raw or 1/2 cup cooked	3-4 times
Brussels Sprouts	1 cup raw or 1/2 cup cooked	2-3 times
Cauliflower	1 cup raw or 1/2 cup cooked	2-3 times
Sweet Potato	1 medium	2-3 times
Carrots	1 medium	2-3 times

Notes:

- Portion sizes are based on typical serving sizes for vegetables.
- Include a variety of colorful vegetables to ensure a broad spectrum of nutrients.

OILS AND FATS

Oils and Fats	Portion Size	Frequency per Week
Olive Oil	1-2 tablespoons	Daily
Flaxseed Oil	1 tablespoon	2-3 times
Walnut Oil	1 tablespoon	2-3 times
Almond Butter	1-2 tablespoons	2-3 times
Avocado	1/2 to 1 medium	3-4 times
Ghee (Clarified Butter)	1-2 tablespoons	1-2 times

Notes:

- Portion sizes are based on typical serving sizes for oils and fats.

- The suggested frequency per week is a general guideline and can be adjusted based on individual preferences and dietary needs.

- Choose high-quality oils, and consider incorporating a variety of fats to ensure a diverse nutrient profile.

CHAPTER 4: BREAKFAST BOOSTERS FOR AB+ INDIVIDUAL

1. Quinoa Berry Breakfast Bowl:

Ingredients:

- 1/2 cup cooked quinoa
- Mixed berries (blueberries, strawberries)
- 1/4 cup Greek yogurt
- Chopped almonds
- Drizzle of honey

Instructions:

1. Mix cooked quinoa with fresh berries.
2. Top with Greek yogurt and chopped almonds.
3. Drizzle honey over the bowl.

2. Avocado and Poached Egg Toast:

Ingredients:

- Whole-grain toast
- Ripe avocado

- Poached egg
- Cherry tomatoes, sliced
- Salt and pepper to taste

Instructions:

1. Smash ripe avocado onto toasted whole-grain bread.

2. Top with a poached egg.

3. Garnish with sliced cherry tomatoes.

4. Season with salt and pepper.

3. Mixed Berry Spinach Smoothie:

Ingredients:

- Mixed berries (strawberries, blueberries, raspberries)
- Handful of spinach leaves
- 1/2 cup Greek yogurt
- 1 tablespoon chia seeds
- Almond milk

Instructions:

1. Blend berries, spinach, Greek yogurt, and almond milk until smooth.

2. Pour into a glass and sprinkle chia seeds on top.

4. Chia Seed Pudding Parfait:

Ingredients:

- Chia seeds
- Almond milk
- Vanilla extract
- Kiwi, mango, berries (fresh fruits)
- Granola

Instructions:

1. Mix chia seeds with almond milk and a splash of vanilla extract.

2. Let it sit in the refrigerator until it thickens.

3. Layer chia seed pudding with fresh fruits and granola.

5. Almond Butter Banana Oatmeal:

Ingredients:

- Rolled oats
- Almond butter
- Sliced banana
- Chopped almonds
- Cinnamon

Instructions:

1. Cook rolled oats according to package instructions.

2. Stir in almond butter.

3. Top with sliced banana, chopped almonds, and a dash of cinnamon.

6. Greek Yogurt and Berry Parfait:

Ingredients:

- Greek yogurt
- Mixed berries (blueberries, strawberries)
- Granola
- Drizzle of honey

Instructions:

1. Layer Greek yogurt with mixed berries.

2. Sprinkle granola on top.

3. Drizzle honey for sweetness.

7. Mango Coconut Chia Pudding:

Ingredients:

- Chia seeds
- Coconut milk
- Fresh mango, diced

- Shredded coconut

Instructions:

1. Mix chia seeds with coconut milk and refrigerate until thickened.

2. Layer with fresh diced mango and shredded coconut.

8. Turkey and Vegetable Omelette:

Ingredients:

- Eggs
- Turkey slices
- Bell peppers, diced
- Spinach leaves
- Feta cheese

Instructions:

1. Whisk eggs and pour into a hot pan.
2. Add turkey, bell peppers, spinach, and feta cheese.
3. Fold the omelette and cook until eggs are set.

9. Blueberry Almond Smoothie Bowl:

Ingredients:

- Frozen blueberries

- Almond milk

- Almond butter

- Banana, sliced

- Granola

Instructions:

1. Blend blueberries, almond milk, and almond butter until smooth.

2. Pour into a bowl and top with sliced banana and granola.

10. Smoked Salmon and Avocado Wrap:

Ingredients:

- Whole-grain wrap

- Smoked salmon

- Avocado slices

- Cream cheese

- Fresh dill

Instructions:

1. Lay smoked salmon on a whole-grain wrap.

2. Add avocado slices, cream cheese, and fresh dill.

3. Roll the wrap and enjoy.

CHAPTER 5: LUNCH DELIGHTS

1. Mediterranean Quinoa Salad:

Ingredients:

- Cooked quinoa
- Cherry tomatoes, halved
- Cucumber, diced
- Kalamata olives, sliced
- Feta cheese, crumbled
- Olive oil
- Lemon juice

Instructions:

1. Combine quinoa, cherry tomatoes, cucumber, olives, and feta cheese.

2. Drizzle with olive oil and lemon juice. Toss well and serve.

2. Turkey and Veggie Stir-Fry:

Ingredients:

- Turkey breast, sliced
- Broccoli florets

Bell peppers, thinly sliced

Snow peas

Garlic, minced

Soy sauce

Sesame oil

Instructions:

1. Stir-fry turkey in sesame oil until cooked.

2. Add garlic, broccoli, bell peppers, and snow peas.

3. Pour soy sauce over the stir-fry and toss until vegetables are tender.

3. Spinach and Feta Stuffed Chicken Breast:

Ingredients:

- Chicken breast
- Fresh spinach leaves
- Feta cheese
- Lemon zest
- Olive oil
- Garlic powder

Instructions:

1. Preheat oven. Butterfly chicken breast.

2. Stuff with spinach, feta, and lemon zest.

3. Drizzle with olive oil, sprinkle with garlic powder, and bake until cooked.

4. Salmon and Quinoa Bowl:

Ingredients:

- Grilled salmon fillet
- Cooked quinoa
- Avocado slices
- Cherry tomatoes, halved
- Cilantro, chopped
- Lime juice

Instructions:

1. Place grilled salmon over a bed of quinoa.

2. Top with avocado slices, cherry tomatoes, and cilantro.

3. Drizzle with lime juice before serving.

5. Vegetarian Chickpea and Spinach Curry:

Ingredients:

- Chickpeas (canned, drained)

- Spinach leaves

- Onion, chopped

- Tomatoes, diced

- Coconut milk

- Curry powder

Instructions:

1. Sauté chopped onions until golden.

2. Add tomatoes, chickpeas, spinach, coconut milk, and curry powder. Simmer until cooked.

6. Greek Salad Wrap:

Ingredients:

- Whole-grain wrap

- Grilled chicken strips

- Cucumber, sliced

- Tomatoes, diced

- Red onion, thinly sliced

- Feta cheese

- Greek dressing

Instructions:

1. Lay chicken strips on a whole-grain wrap.

2. Add cucumber, tomatoes, red onion, and feta.

3. Drizzle with Greek dressing, wrap, and enjoy.

7. Stuffed Bell Peppers with Quinoa and Black Beans:

Ingredients:

Bell peppers, halved

Cooked quinoa

Black beans (canned, drained)

Corn kernels

Salsa

Shredded cheese

Instructions:

1. Mix quinoa, black beans, corn, and salsa.

2. Stuff bell peppers with the mixture.

3. Top with shredded cheese and bake until peppers are tender.

8. Sesame Ginger Tofu Stir-Fry:

Ingredients:

- Extra-firm tofu, cubed
- Broccoli florets
- Carrots, julienned
- Snap peas
- Sesame oil
- Ginger, minced
- Low-sodium soy sauce

Instructions:

1. Sauté tofu in sesame oil until golden.

2. Add ginger, broccoli, carrots, and snap peas.

3. Pour soy sauce over the stir-fry and toss until vegetables are cooked.

9. Caprese Salad with Balsamic Glaze:

Ingredients:

- Fresh mozzarella, sliced
- Tomatoes, sliced
- Fresh basil leaves
- Balsamic glaze
- Olive oil

- Salt and pepper to taste

Instructions:

1. Arrange mozzarella, tomatoes, and basil on a plate.

2. Drizzle with balsamic glaze and olive oil.

3. Season with salt and pepper.

10. Lentil and Vegetable Soup:

Ingredients:

- Lentils (dry, rinsed)

- Carrots, diced

- Celery, chopped

- Onion, diced

- Garlic, minced

- Vegetable broth

- Italian seasoning

Instructions:

1. Sauté onions and garlic until fragrant.

2. Add lentils, carrots, celery, vegetable broth, and Italian seasoning.

3. Simmer until lentils are tender.

CHAPTER 6: DINNER INDULGENCES

1. Salmon with Lemon-Dill Sauce:

Ingredients:

- Salmon fillets
- Lemon juice
- Fresh dill, chopped
- Olive oil
- Garlic powder

Instructions:

1. Preheat the oven. Place salmon on a baking sheet.

2. Mix lemon juice, chopped dill, olive oil, and garlic powder.

3. Brush the mixture over salmon and bake until cooked.

2. Vegetarian Quinoa Stuffed Bell Peppers:

Ingredients:

- Bell peppers, halved
- Cooked quinoa

- Black beans (canned, drained)

- Corn kernels

- Diced tomatoes

- Cumin and chili powder

Instructions:

1. Mix quinoa, black beans, corn, diced tomatoes, cumin, and chili powder.

2. Stuff bell peppers with the mixture and bake until peppers are tender.

3. Grilled Chicken and Vegetable Skewers:

Ingredients:

- Chicken breast, cut into cubes

- Bell peppers, cherry tomatoes, red onion

- Olive oil

- Lemon juice

- Oregano and garlic powder

Instructions:

1. Thread chicken and vegetables onto skewers.

2. Mix olive oil, lemon juice, oregano, and garlic powder for a marinade.

3. Grill skewers until chicken is cooked.

4. Mushroom and Spinach Stuffed Chicken Breast:

Ingredients:

- Chicken breast

- Mushrooms, chopped

- Fresh spinach

- Goat cheese

- Garlic, minced

Instructions:

1. Sauté mushrooms and garlic until cooked.

2. Stuff chicken breast with sautéed mushrooms, fresh spinach, and goat cheese.

3. Bake until chicken is cooked through.

5. Shrimp and Broccoli Stir-Fry:

Ingredients:

- Shrimp, peeled and deveined

- Broccoli florets
- Bell peppers, sliced
- Ginger and garlic, minced
- Soy sauce
- Sesame oil

Instructions:

1. Sauté shrimp, broccoli, and bell peppers in sesame oil.

2. Add minced ginger and garlic.

3. Pour soy sauce over the stir-fry and cook until shrimp is pink.

6. Eggplant and Chickpea Curry:

Ingredients:

- Eggplant, diced
- Chickpeas (canned, drained)
- Coconut milk
- Curry powder
- Turmeric and cumin

Instructions:

1. Cook eggplant until softened.

2. Add chickpeas, coconut milk, curry powder, turmeric, and cumin.

3. Simmer until flavors meld.

7. Baked Cod with Mediterranean Salsa:

Ingredients:

- Cod fillets
- Tomatoes, diced
- Cucumber, diced
- Red onion, finely chopped
- Kalamata olives, sliced
- Olive oil
- Fresh parsley, chopped

Instructions:

1. Place cod fillets on a baking sheet.

2. Mix diced tomatoes, cucumber, red onion, olives, olive oil, and fresh parsley.

3. Top cod with the salsa and bake until fish is cooked.

8. Turkey and Quinoa Stuffed Acorn Squash:

Ingredients:

- Acorn squash, halved
- Ground turkey
- Cooked quinoa
- Diced apples
- Sage and thyme

Instructions:

1. Roast acorn squash until tender.

2. Sauté ground turkey, cooked quinoa, diced apples, sage, and thyme.

3. Stuff acorn squash with the turkey-quinoa mixture.

9. Lentil and Vegetable Stir-Fry:

Ingredients:

- Cooked lentils
- Broccoli florets
- Carrots, julienned
- Bell peppers, sliced
- Soy sauce

- Sesame oil

Instructions:

1. Sauté vegetables in sesame oil until tender.

2. Add cooked lentils and soy sauce.

3. Stir-fry until heated through.

10. Chickpea and Spinach Coconut Curry:

Ingredients:

- Chickpeas (canned, drained)
- Fresh spinach
- Coconut milk
- Curry powder
- Garlic and ginger, minced

Instructions:

1. Sauté garlic and ginger until fragrant.

2. Add chickpeas, fresh spinach, coconut milk, and curry powder.

3. Simmer until flavors meld.

CHAPTER 7: SNACKS AND SWEETS

1. Greek Yogurt and Berry Parfait:

Ingredients:

- Greek yogurt
- Mixed berries (blueberries, strawberries)
- Granola
- Drizzle of honey

Instructions:

1. Layer Greek yogurt with mixed berries.
2. Sprinkle granola on top.
3. Drizzle with honey for sweetness.

2. Almond Butter and Banana Rice Cakes:

Ingredients:

- Rice cakes
- Almond butter
- Banana, sliced
- Chia seeds

Instructions:

1. Spread almond butter on rice cakes.

2. Top with banana slices and sprinkle chia seeds.

3. Roasted Chickpeas with Herbs:

Ingredients:

- Chickpeas (canned, drained)
- Olive oil
- Garlic powder, cumin, and paprika

Instructions:

1. Toss chickpeas with olive oil and spices.

2. Roast until crispy.

4. Fruit Kabobs with Mint Yogurt Dip:

Ingredients:

- Assorted fruits (grapes, melon, pineapple)
- Wooden skewers
- Greek yogurt
- Fresh mint, chopped

- Honey

Instructions:

1. Thread assorted fruits onto skewers.

2. Mix Greek yogurt with chopped mint and honey for a dipping sauce.

5. Dark Chocolate-Dipped Strawberries:

Ingredients:

- Strawberries, washed and dried
- Dark chocolate (70% cocoa or higher)

Instructions:

1. Melt dark chocolate.

2. Dip each strawberry into the melted chocolate.

3. Place on a parchment paper-lined tray to cool.

6. Trail Mix with Nuts and Dried Fruits:

Ingredients:

- Almonds, walnuts, cashews

- Dried cranberries

- Pumpkin seeds

- Dark chocolate chips

Instructions:

1. Mix nuts, dried cranberries, pumpkin seeds, and dark chocolate chips.

2. Portion into snack-sized servings.

7. Avocado Chocolate Mousse:

Ingredients:

- Ripe avocados

- Cocoa powder

- Maple syrup or honey

- Vanilla extract

Instructions:

1. Blend avocados, cocoa powder, maple syrup (or honey), and vanilla extract until smooth.

2. Chill before serving.

8. Mango Salsa with Cinnamon Tortilla Chips:

Ingredients:

- Mango, diced
- Red onion, finely chopped
- Jalapeño, minced
- Fresh cilantro, chopped
- Whole-grain tortillas
- Cinnamon

Instructions:

1. Mix mango, red onion, jalapeño, and cilantro for salsa.

2. Cut tortillas into wedges, sprinkle with cinnamon, and bake until crisp.

9. Chia Seed Pudding with Almond Milk:

Ingredients:

- Chia seeds
- Almond milk
- Vanilla extract
- Fresh berries for topping

Instructions:

1. Mix chia seeds with almond milk and vanilla extract.

2. Refrigerate until thickened.

3. Top with fresh berries before serving.

10. Coconut Energy Bites:

Ingredients:

- Shredded coconut
- Almond flour
- Medjool dates, pitted
- Almond butter

Instructions:

1. Blend shredded coconut, almond flour, dates, and almond butter until a dough forms.

2. Roll into small bites and refrigerate.

CHAPTER 8: BEVERAGES WITH A BOOST

1. Green Detox Smoothie:

Ingredients:

- Spinach
- Cucumber
- Kiwi
- Green apple
- Chia seeds
- Almond milk

Instructions:

1. Blend spinach, cucumber, kiwi, green apple, and chia seeds.

2. Add almond milk and blend until smooth.

2. Berry Blast Smoothie:

Ingredients:

- Mixed berries (blueberries, strawberries, raspberries)
- Banana

- Greek yogurt
- Almond milk
- Ice cubes

Instructions:

1. Blend mixed berries, banana, Greek yogurt, and almond milk.

2. Add ice cubes and blend until creamy.

3. Tropical Paradise Smoothie:

Ingredients:

- Pineapple chunks
- Mango
- Coconut water
- Fresh lime juice
- Mint leaves

Instructions:

1. Blend pineapple, mango, coconut water, lime juice, and mint leaves.

2. Serve over ice.

4. Protein-Packed Almond Butter Smoothie:

Ingredients:

- Almond butter
- Banana
- Protein powder
- Almond milk
- Flaxseeds

Instructions:

1. Blend almond butter, banana, protein powder, and almond milk.

2. Add flaxseeds for an extra boost.

5. Cherry Almond Chia Smoothie:

Ingredients:

- Cherries (frozen or fresh)
- Almond milk
- Almond extract
- Chia seeds
- Honey (optional)

Instructions:

1. Blend cherries, almond milk, almond extract, and chia seeds.

2. Add honey for sweetness if desired.

6. Coconut Ginger Zinger:

Ingredients:

- Coconut water
- Pineapple
- Ginger
- Lime
- Fresh mint leaves

Instructions:

1. Blend coconut water, pineapple, ginger, and lime.

2. Add fresh mint leaves and blend until smooth.

7. Cucumber Mint Cooler:

Ingredients:

- Cucumber
- Mint leaves
- Lime juice
- Honey

- Ice cubes

Instructions:

1. Blend cucumber, mint leaves, lime juice, and honey.

2. Serve over ice for a refreshing drink.

8. Pomegranate Blueberry Bliss:

Ingredients:

- Pomegranate seeds
- Blueberries
- Greek yogurt
- Almond milk
- Flaxseeds

Instructions:

1. Blend pomegranate seeds, blueberries, Greek yogurt, and almond milk.

2. Add flaxseeds for extra nutrition.

9. Citrus Sunshine Smoothie:

Ingredients:

- Oranges
- Pineapple

- Greek yogurt

- Coconut milk

- Turmeric

Instructions:

1. Blend oranges, pineapple, Greek yogurt, coconut milk, and a pinch of turmeric.

2. Enjoy this vibrant citrus smoothie.

10. Vanilla Matcha Latte:

Ingredients:

Matcha powder

Almond milk

Vanilla extract

Honey

Instructions:

1. Whisk matcha powder with a small amount of hot water until smooth.

2. Heat almond milk, add vanilla extract, and pour over the matcha.

3. Sweeten with honey to taste.

14-DAY MEAL PLAN FOR AB+ INDIVIDUAL

WEEK 1

Day 1:

- **Breakfast:** Quinoa Berry Breakfast Bowl
- **Lunch:** Mediterranean Quinoa Salad
- **Dinner:** Salmon with Lemon-Dill Sauce
- **Snack:** Greek Yogurt and Berry Parfait

Day 2:

- **Breakfast:** Avocado and Poached Egg Toast
- **Lunch:** Vegetarian Chickpea and Spinach Curry
- **Dinner:** Grilled Chicken and Vegetable Skewers
- **Snack:** Almond Butter and Banana Rice Cakes

Day 3:

- **Breakfast:** Mixed Berry Spinach Smoothie
- **Lunch:** Stuffed Bell Peppers with Quinoa and Black Beans

- **Dinner:** Mushroom and Spinach Stuffed Chicken Breast
- **Snack:** Roasted Chickpeas with Herbs

Day 4:

- **Breakfast:** Chia Seed Pudding Parfait
- **Lunch:** Greek Salad Wrap
- **Dinner:** Baked Cod with Mediterranean Salsa
- **Snack:** Fruit Kabobs with Mint Yogurt Dip

Day 5:

- **Breakfast:** Almond Butter Banana Oatmeal
- **Lunch:** Lentil and Vegetable Stir-Fry
- **Dinner:** Shrimp and Broccoli Stir-Fry
- **Snack:** Dark Chocolate-Dipped Strawberries

Day 6:

- **Breakfast:** Mango Coconut Chia Pudding
- **Lunch:** Caprese Salad with Balsamic Glaze
- **Dinner:** Eggplant and Chickpea Curry
- **Snack:** Trail Mix with Nuts and Dried Fruits

Day 7:

- **Breakfast:** Blueberry Almond Smoothie Bowl
- **Lunch:** Sesame Ginger Tofu Stir-Fry
- **Dinner:** Turkey and Quinoa Stuffed Acorn Squash
- **Snack:** Avocado Chocolate Mousse

WEEK 2

Day 8:

- **Breakfast:** Smoked Salmon and Avocado Wrap
- **Lunch:** Stuffed Bell Peppers with Quinoa and Black Beans
- **Dinner:** Lentil and Vegetable Soup
- **Snack:** Coconut Energy Bites

Day 9:

- **Breakfast:** Greek Yogurt and Berry Parfait
- **Lunch:** Chickpea and Spinach Coconut Curry
- **Dinner:** Vegetarian Quinoa Stuffed Bell Peppers
- **Snack:** Almond Butter and Banana Rice Cakes

Day 10:

- **Breakfast:** Quinoa Berry Breakfast Bowl
- **Lunch:** Mediterranean Quinoa Salad
- **Dinner:** Salmon with Lemon-Dill Sauce
- **Snack:** Roasted Chickpeas with Herbs

Day 11:

- **Breakfast:** Avocado and Poached Egg Toast
- **Lunch:** Greek Salad Wrap
- **Dinner:** Grilled Chicken and Vegetable Skewers
- **Snack:** Dark Chocolate-Dipped Strawberries

Day 12:

- **Breakfast:** Mixed Berry Spinach Smoothie
- **Lunch:** Mushroom and Spinach Stuffed Chicken Breast
- **Dinner:** Shrimp and Broccoli Stir-Fry
- **Snack:** Fruit Kabobs with Mint Yogurt Dip

Day 13:

- **Breakfast:** Chia Seed Pudding Parfait
- **Lunch:** Caprese Salad with Balsamic Glaze

- **Dinner:** Eggplant and Chickpea Curry

- **Snack:** Trail Mix with Nuts and Dried Fruits

Day 14:

- **Breakfast:** Blueberry Almond Smoothie Bowl

- **Lunch:** Sesame Ginger Tofu Stir-Fry

- **Dinner:** Turkey and Quinoa Stuffed Acorn Squash

- **Snack:** Coconut Energy Bites

CONCLUSION

In concluding the **"Blood Type AB Positive Diet Book,"** our culinary journey has been more than a collection of recipes; it's a celebration of well-being tailored specifically for individuals with Blood Type AB+. We've explored the diverse and flavorful realm of foods that resonate harmoniously with your unique physiology, aiming not just for nourishment but for a holistic approach to health.

Through these pages, we've witnessed the transformative power of mindful eating, providing not only physical sustenance but also fostering a profound connection between your plate and your well-being. By embracing the recommended ingredients and culinary practices, you've embarked on a personalized and sustainable path towards a healthier lifestyle.

The personal stories shared within these chapters serve as testaments to the positive impact this cookbook can have. From heightened energy levels to an improved sense of vitality, readers have embraced the idea that food can be both medicine and pleasure.

As you continue to experiment with these recipes, remember that your health journey is unique, and small changes can yield significant results. Consult with healthcare professionals for personalized guidance and listen to your body as it thrives on the nourishing and delicious choices laid out in this cookbook. Here's to your continued well-being and the joyous exploration of a blood type-conscious culinary adventure!